MANAGE YOUR MEDICAL CONDITION

Dr. Talya Miron-Shatz and the Buddy&Soul team

INTRODUCTION: WELCOME TO MANAGING YOUR MEDICAL CONDITION

Being diagnosed with a medical condition is just the start. It marks the beginning of a journey into the unknown. And, whether you like it or not, on this journey, you are the captain of that boat! Or at least, the co-captain, alongside your physician. Because, let's face it, there are very few situations in which your involvement is not at all required. Even by opening your mouth to swallow a pill.

Maybe you're one of those people who like to take charge, assume responsibility, and be very involved with what is going on. Or maybe, at a time like this, you would much rather move over to the passenger seat. Either way, we are living at a fantastic age, where the variety and accessibility of medical information allows for patients to take charge over their health. And [science shows](#) that patients who participate in decision making achieve better medical outcomes. So actively managing your health is both a viable and beneficial option, which, even if you don't like, you must seriously consider.

It's not simple. In so many ways. Not only is it emotionally draining to be ill, it is also mentally perplexing. I should know. Most of my academic career, and most of my publications, have been around the ways patients understand medical information. Repeatedly, I found that patients, and people in general, want to make informed choices and are unable to because of the inundation of confusing medical information. They end up making decisions based upon attitudes and preconceptions that are actually worse for them. Ironically, whenever I am a patient, I find myself making the same mistakes, along with many others.

This course is intended to help put things in order, to prevent you from making obvious mistakes, and to give you some tools for becoming actively involved with managing your health, to the degree you are comfortable with. You can practice it alone, or with someone you trust, who cares enough to participate. Hope this helps you navigate your boat safely back to health.

There are three goals that we had in mind while creating this book. We want you to:

- Gain tools to actively manage your health.
- Learn how to sort through and interpret medical information.
- Assume responsibility for how you manage your medical condition.

There are so many unknowns when it comes to illness and disease. It's easy to throw your hands up and say, "I'll leave it up to the doctors!" But patient advocacy and involvement have been scientifically proven to produce higher levels of satisfaction and better health outcomes. This course will help you take control of and manage your condition, whether acute or chronic.

YOUR JOURNEY TO MANAGING YOUR MEDICAL CONDITION

INTRODUCTION: Welcome to Manage Your Medical Condition .... Page 2

How To Use This Book .... Page 4

Why I Created Buddy&Soul .... Page 5

STRATEGY 1: Write a Medical Mission Statement .... Page 8

STRATEGY 2: Organize your Medical Clutter .... Page 15

STRATEGY 3: Do your Math .... Page 22

STRATEGY 4: Get Real about your Condition .... Page 29

STRATEGY 5: Assume Responsibility .... Page 36

STRATEGY 6: Evaluate your Choices .... Page 43

STRATEGY 7: Get your Body on Track .... Page 50

STRATEGY 8: Forget your Condition for a Change .... Page 57

STRATEGY 9: Get the Help you Need .... Page 64

STRATEGY 10: Check your Checklist .... Page 71

Where Do We Go From Here .... Page 78

HOW TO USE THIS BOOK TO MANAGE YOUR MEDICAL CONDITION

In this book you'll find ten great strategies for achieving the goals we listed above. You'll also find inspiring content and exercises you can engage with to help you practice emotionally managing your illness. You will get the most out of this book by going through the strategies and associated exercises one by one. Of course, you can also simply read it the whole way through. But we recommend using this book by going through it in order, watching the TED talks, and doing the exercises. We have found the best way to do the exercises is by dedicating a notebook as your course journal. If you're reading this book on a PC, feel free to create a text file and use that as your course journal. Or you could simply use a good ol' pen and paper to do the exercises. Either way, we recommend keeping some method of writing handy while you go through the exercises in this book to optimize what you get out of it.

To maximize your experience with the Buddy and Soul book, share your thoughts and insights with us on social media! Post pictures relating to your progress on Instagram and Twitter, tagging @Buddy_N_Soul, and Facebook @Buddy&Soul. By sharing with us on social media, not only can you help others with their personal journeys, you can read about those facing similar challenges.

Direct message us YOUR story @Buddy_N_Soul on Instagram and be anonymously featured for a chance to **win a Buddy&Soul three month free membership**.

If you really want to go all the way, visit our website, BuddynSoul.com, and explore all that we have to offer beyond 'Manage your Medical Condition'. In fact, we have two other books in the Medical Series that we think you might benefit from: Emotionally Managing Your Illness and Adhering to Your Medication

WHY I CREATED BUDDY&SOUL AND WHY I CREATED THIS BOOK

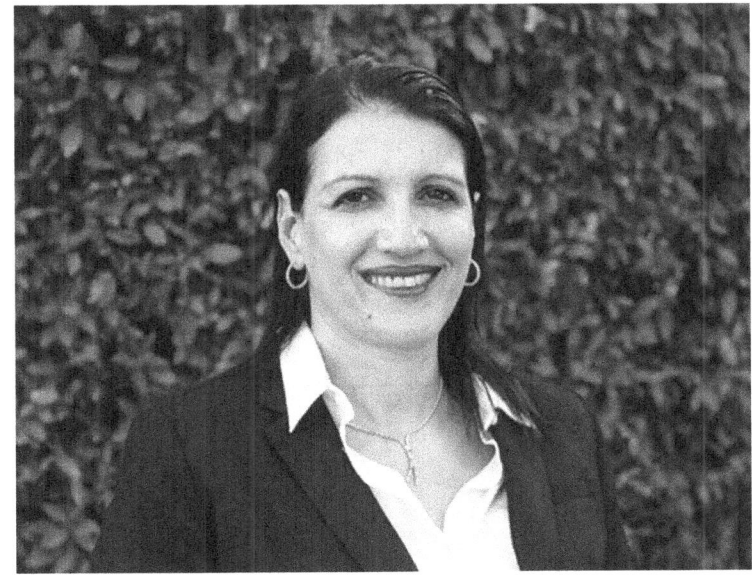

I'm Dr. Talya Miron-Shatz, CEO of Buddy&Soul, where Emotionally Managing Your Illness and many more e-courses and books come from. I have a PhD in psychology and was very fortunate to do my post-doc at Princeton University with Nobel Laureate Daniel Kahneman. I've also taught at the Wharton Business School, University of Pennsylvania. Now I'm a professor at the Ono Academic College, and a visiting researcher at Cambridge University. I used to study happiness, and for a long time now, I've been studying medical decision making and helping organizations support people on their way to joy and health. One thing that struck me as unfair was that we were expecting people to change their life for good but weren't giving them the tools to do so. People deserve all the help they can get when breaking out of old patterns and moving their lives forward.

This is what Buddy&Soul does.

We support you in many ways by providing science-based actionable ways to sustain your body and mind. We help you sleep better, spark a change in your eating habits, and manage stress. We teach you how to create new habits and how to engage your willpower. We help you grow, claim your self-esteem, cultivate authenticity, reframe your life story, achieve your goals and so much more including

Everything you need to change your life for good.

I want to hear from YOU! Please feel free to send me an email with your thoughts, suggestions, and feedback regarding this book to talya@buddynsoul.com. I would love to hear what you think about this book and how it helped you with managing your medical condition. Your feedback is extremely valuable and will allow us to help more individuals, like yourself, to obtain the necessary tools and support needed to change their lives for good.

What do you hope to gain from Manage Your Medical Condition?

There is so much to gain with any action that you take towards improving your medical condition. Knowledge, state of mind and being well informed can be just as important as the techniques and treatments themselves.

1. The positive reinforcement will improve my health.
2. I'll learn about techniques and methods I didn't know were out there.
3. Joining a community of people that are going through the same thing as me.
4. A feeling of being proactive with my medical condition.
5. Hope.

Add your own:

6. _____

7. _____

8. _____

5 Tips to keep you motivated through Manage Your Medical Condition

It's easy to get discouraged with just about anything in life. Managing a medical condition is no different. Be proactive in building up motivational momentum and keeping it going. Be your own best resource by producing reminders of your motivation for when you need them the most.

Keep a picture of your loved ones near you at all times. Look at it whenever you need the most motivation.

1. Create a network of people who have gone through what you're going through. Turn to one or more of them whenever you're feeling discouraged.
2. Write a daily gratitude journal of at least three things you're grateful for. This should be the last thing you do before going to bed. You'll find that even on the hardest days you'll have things to be grateful for.
3. Whenever you find yourself feeling positive, write a note to yourself to remind you of that feeling when you need it the most. You can also record yourself an audio or video message.
4. Take matters into your own hands by doing research. Become as familiar as possible with your medical condition. Discuss your findings with your doctor to make sure you have a good grasp on the science behind what you're dealing with.
5. Make a list of things you wished someone had told you before you started dealing with your medical condition. Share this with people who haven't been dealing with the medical condition as long as you have.

Strategy 1: Write a medical mission statement

If you've ever read *The 7 Habits of Highly Effective People,* you'll be familiar with Stephen Covey's claim that "all things are created twice."

In the first creation, you draw the blueprints, write the speech, or map out your route; in the second you make thing happen – build that building, give the speech, or take your road trip.

Covey's amazing insight is that success and failure are often determined *before* you even begin putting plans into practice. In his words, "Most business failures begin in the first creation, with problems such as undercapitalization, misunderstanding of the market, or lack of a business plan" (p. 99).

If Covey is right and success really starts in the planning stages, then why should managing a medical condition be any different?

With this in mind, before delving deep into the nitty-gritty of meds, diet, paperwork, etc., let's invest in the stage of first creation.

Write a medical mission statement that clearly spells out where you're headed and what you're hoping to accomplish with this course.

Ask yourself some fundamental questions: What would it look like to successfully manage your condition? What would it mean in terms of your meds, your daily routines, your diet, or any lifestyle changes you'd need to make? In what areas would you have to become more knowledgeable? How would you be able to gauge your progress?

You can make it specific – 'Keeping my BMI below 25 and filling my prescriptions on time' – or broad – 'Being informed and on top of what my condition means and what managing it requires.'

In either case, getting *something* down in writing will both help you keep focused throughout the course and create a greater sense of commitment to your medical goals.

Remember, what you're working towards here is totally personal and no two medical mission statements will look alike. There are no rights or wrongs. The point is for you to feel this statement represents who you are and what's important to you.

EXERCISE

Craft your medical mission statement in your journal now. Ask yourself where you'd like to be by the end of the course, and get writing.

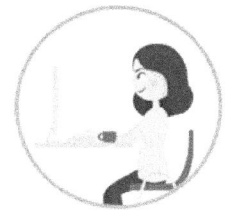

TIPS

Tip 1: There are as many ways to write a personal mission statement as there are people in the world, so there's really no way you can get it wrong!

Tip 2: This will be available for your reference as you proceed with the rest of the course... and beyond.

Tip 3: For help with goal setting check out our Achieve Your Goals course.

DRIVING THE MESSAGE HOME

I'm glad that you've decided to join us for the Manage Your Medical Condition course. Each session of our course consists of a warm-up talk, followed by a hands-on component where you'll learn a new skill or idea and have a chance to start putting it into action.

Our first session in Manage Your Medical Condition is about setting some goals for the course. Before we get to that, though, let's take a moment to meet Aimee Mullins, who was born without shinbones, and at a young age had both her lower legs amputated. While others may label her disabled, Mullins chooses to frame her condition as an adversity rather than an illness. She is a known athlete, actress, and model. Human potential should not be limited by what others determine you are able to achieve. Mullins empowers those of us who suffer from a medical condition and have been made to feel limited or lacking in some way because of it. An important element to keep in mind as you'll soon be asked to create a medical mission statement.

We think you'll find that the more you put into the course, the more you'll get out of it. So take full advantage of all our features and find your place in a community of people facing similar challenges.

Watch 'The Opportunity of Adversity' presented by Aimee Mullins on YouTube.

What are your most pressing medical goals?

Setting goals is a great way to stay on track and ensure you accomplish your dreams for the future. What are some of your goals when it comes to your medical condition?

(Plus: Check out our Achieve Your Goals course)

1. To better adhere to my medication
2. To become a more informed patient
3. To build a better alliance with my doctors
4. To stop turning to Dr. Google all the time
5. To take ownership of my treatment course
6. To invest more time in me as a person and not a medical condition

Add your own:

7. _____

8. _____

9. _____

Can a mission statement actually impact my health?

Writing a medical mission statement sounds like a good idea...if you've got nothing better to do with your time. But c'mon. I'm busy taking care of my medical condition here. I have more pressing priorities than that!

For:

1. A mission statement is just what I need. It will help me clarify my focus and give me direction.
2. By putting my hopes and dreams about my medical condition into words, I'll be much more likely to strive to accomplish them.
3. I'm not goal-oriented and a medical mission statement is a great tool to help me get more goal-focused.

Add your own argument:

4. _____

Against:

1. It's nice to have direction but if you have limited time and resources, it's definitely not #1 on the to-do list.
2. Words are meaningless. It's actions that matter.
3. A medical mission statement will make me feel bad about myself if I fail to live up to it. I don't need that kind of pressure.

Add your own argument:

4. _____

TAKE A FEW MINUTES AND WRITE IN YOUR COURSE JOURNAL...

The hardest part about writing a medical mission statement

It might be hard to tease apart the various goals you have for this course. Share with the community what's holding you back from successfully outlining how you wish to succeed with this course, and perhaps receive insights from others facing similar challenges.

Take some time brainstorming in your journal about your experience with your medical condition, and then share your story with the Buddy and Soul community! Tag us on Instagram and Twitter @Buddy_N_Soul, using the **#BuddynSoulMedSupport**. You can also direct message us YOUR story @Buddy_N_Soul on Instagram and be anonymously featured for a chance to **win a Buddy&Soul three month free membership**. By sharing with us on social media, not only can you help others with their personal journeys, you can read about those facing similar challenges.

Embracing adversity doesn't apply to a medical condition.

In Aimee Mullins' TED Talk *The Opportunity of Adversity*, she shares the power of reframing adversity as an opportunity. That's nice for Mullins, but I'm a different person, dealing with different condition. Her message can't possibly apply to me!
(Plus: Check out our Everyday Reframing course)

For:

1. What Mullins says can apply to all medical conditions, and in fact, all tough situations in life. There is always opportunity to be found within.
2. Yes, for some people and with some conditions it might be harder to find the opportunity that Mullins describes, but it's never impossible.

Add your own argument:

3. _____

Against:

1. Her message is based on a disability and I'm dealing with an illness.
2. My medical condition will hopefully be temporary and then I'll be back to my normal self. We're talking apples and oranges.

Add your own argument:

3. _____

Strategy 2: Organize your medical clutter

With illness comes an abundance of…papers! (Which nowadays also means digital files.) From every doctor comes a seemingly endless stream of medication pamphlets, reports, lab results, insurance papers and much more. Some of this paperwork shows up in your inbox where you can more readily store it without contributing to the clutterfest. However, much of this paperwork is physically handed to you and can now be found in the most random of corners of your home.

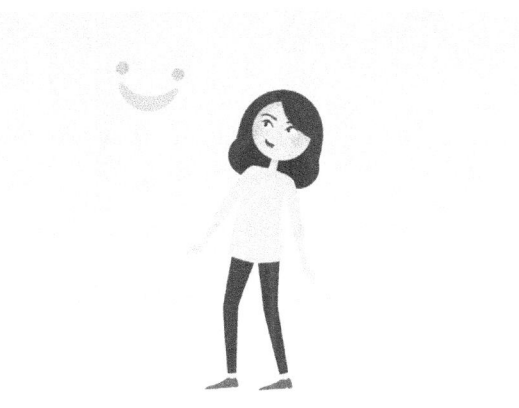

Rather than searching for a spoon and chancing upon your insurance receipt, or taking a nap on the couch only to find your missing lab results between the cushions, better rein it in and preempt a clutter attack down the line.

Judith Rodin, associate professor at Yale University and president of the Rockefeller Foundation, writes in the *Handbook of the Psychology of Aging* about the importance of control when it comes to illness. "Interventions to enhance feelings of control in elderly people have shown substantial improvements in health" (p. 139). In fact, it is the feeling of a loss of control that contributes to the elderly getting sick more quickly.

The same principle presumably holds true for anyone managing a medical condition: a sense of control leads to better health.

To regain at least a semblance of control amid all the unknowns and unknowables of a medical condition, **take some time to organize your papers. A small step, but far from trivial!**

This involves determining:

    1. **Where** you want to keep your files. Are you going to put them in an accordion file, a specific drawer, or digitalize your documents?
    2. **How** you want to organize your files. Is it going to be according to content, dates, color? Whatever helps you stay organized.
    3. **Whom** you want to be in charge of keeping up your medical files. You? Your partner? Your super-organized brother-in-law?

Give yourself honest responses, based on your organizational skills. If you're a messier type, then getting all your medical papers into one bag or folder will already be an improvement. And if you could separate to 'insurance' and 'medical,' all the better.

The more specific the answers you give, the more likely this is to actually happen.
Whether it means buying an accordion folder, designating a drawer in your house, or taking pictures of everything on your smartphone and ditching the hard copies altogether, get your paperwork – and your medical condition – under control ASAP.

EXERCISE

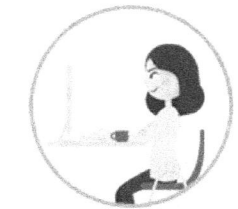

Step 1: Right now, start yourself off by answering the three questions we mentioned before in your journal:

1. **Where** do you plan to keep your medical papers?
2. **How** will you organize them?
3. **Who** will be in charge of keeping your folders up-to-date and organized on a regular basis?

Step 2: Dedicate some time this week to getting your medical paperwork sorted. **Schedule it into your calendar right now.**

TIPS

Tip 1: Boast a bit! For bonus points come back when you're done and upload a picture of your finished – and very organized – medical folder.

Tip 2: Not the organized type? Elicit help from someone who is. Your friends and family want to help you. Here's their chance.

Tip 3: If you go the folder route, buy a bright color. Don't go for anything grim that will give you the wrong feeling whenever you look at it.

Tip 4: For tools on how to turn organization from a burst of inspiration into a habit, check out our Habit Workshop course.

Tip 5: Not sure what type of organizer you are? Check out our Cultivating Authenticity course to learn more about who *you* are.

DRIVING THE MESSAGE HOME

We've chosen a talk for today's session that will hopefully convince you that when it comes to clutter and papers, less is really more.

We live in a big consumer world where the message is: have more to be more. We need to have bigger houses, more money, and more stuff. But what kind of impact does that have on our health?

As you watch, ask yourself where you could declutter or minimize, especially on the medical clutter front. What would happen if – like David Friedlander in the clip we're about to see – you took on the perspective of less is more?

Following the clip, you'll be given the opportunity to go ahead and do some of your own decluttering. We think and hope you'll find it makes a big difference in managing your medical condition.

Watch 'Less- The Lifestyle' presented by David Friedlander at TEDxDumbo on YouTube.

Can organizing my papers really help my medical condition?

There are plenty of things to do when you are trying to manage your illness. Is organization really that integral?

For:

1. If I'm organized then I won't be wasting time trying to find important documents. I save time in the long run.
2. Organization gives me a sense of control – completely priceless when I'm sick.
3. I feel a lot of anxiety when my surroundings are a mess. Having paperwork all over the place is simply stressful.
4. I need to take responsibility for my illness. Organizing my paperwork is part of it.

Add your own argument:

5. _____

Against:

1. I am limited in my time and resources. The more I expend myself organizing my swag, the less available I'll be to manage the illness itself.
2. I like the mess. Every time I need a paper, it's like "Medical File Find, Extreme Edition."
3. When you're in survival mode, there's no need for organization.
4. Organizing my papers is something I can easily designate to someone else. I don't have to be in charge of it.

Add your own argument:

5. _____

What motivates you to keep your medical files organized?

We all know what it takes to organize a never-ending amount of papers, and it's not easy! What helps you stay organized when you're managing an illness?

1. Nothing! I designate organization to someone else.
2. A little bit at a time. That way it's not overwhelming.
3. I just do it! I don't stop until I'm finished.
4. I think about getting better. I'll do anything to get better.
5. I like to have things organized. It makes me feel more in control.

Add your own:

6. _____

7. _____

8. _____

Take some time brainstorming in your journal about your experience with your medical condition, and then share your story with the Buddy and Soul community! Tag us on Instagram and Twitter @Buddy_N_Soul, using the **#BuddynSoulMedSupport**. By sharing with us on social media, not only can you help others with their personal journeys, you can read about those facing similar challenges.

TAKE A FEW MINUTES AND WRITE IN YOUR COURSE JOURNAL...

How I got my medical clutter under control

The shift from "big bag full of documents, receipts, test results, and rubbish" to "a normal folder with what I need" is an amazing move, but not magic. Share with the community how you were able to make that shift, and maybe help others who are struggling with a similar challenge.

Direct message us YOUR story @Buddy_N_Soul on Instagram and be anonymously featured for a chance to **win a Buddy&Soul three month free membership**.

9 Ways decluttering can help you manage your health

You don't always have complete control over your health. Something you do have control over, however, is the level of clutter and organization in your life. Advocates of minimalism believe that your health and wellbeing are fundamentally intertwined with your surroundings. Here's why.

1. Your health is a priority. Focusing on quality over quantity will leave you with fewer distractions and frustrations.
2. Your home is your safe space. Let it reflect how you want to feel on the inside.
3. Becoming more efficient and better organized in your daily life will help you to also be more efficient and better organized with things related to your health.
4. Organizing and consolidating will help take your mind off of things like your health problems. The more headspace your health takes up, the more frustrating it will be for you. Declutter your mind as well as your living space.
(Plus: Check out our Declutter Your Mind course)
5. With less things in your life you'll have less things to worry about.
6. Becoming better at deciding what you need versus what you want will teach you to better prioritize your health (and your life).

Add your own:

7. _____

8. _____

9. _____

Take some time brainstorming in your journal about your experience with your medical condition, and then share your story with the Buddy and Soul community! Tag us on Instagram and Twitter @Buddy_N_Soul, using the **#BuddynSoulMedSupport**. By sharing with us on social media, not only can you help others with their personal journeys, you can read about those facing similar challenges.

Strategy 3: Do your math

The title of this session might read as an insult. I can assure you it is not. I spent the better part of my academic career studying how people understand medical information, and realizing they often get it wrong. It is not their fault, by the way. If information is unintelligible to about 50% of the population, then we either need to replace the population, or the way information is presented.

Probabilities, in particular, are vicious. They seem so innocuous but are so often misinterpreted.

Just as an anecdote, my PhD student was a genetic counselor. A woman coming for consultation had a 1:92 chance of having a baby with Down syndrome. The counselor explained it was just over 1% chance, to which the woman responded, "That's all?! I thought it was 8%." How on earth did she get to 8%? She knew there could only be 100% of something, so she subtracted the 92 from 100, coming up with 8.

A more scientific example comes from a study some colleagues and I published in *Judgment and Decision Making*. We took information from the National Cancer Institute about BRCA gene mutations, the gene associated with breast and ovarian cancer. Women who carry the gene mutation have a 60% chance of developing breast cancer. Almost half of our participants falsely interpreted this statistic to mean that women who carry the BRCA gene had a "60% higher chance" of developing cancer (p. 116).

The good news is that knowing how to ask good questions is more than half the battle when it comes to managing your illness.

In particular, asking your doctor to restate numbers using the frequentist format – where instead of percentages you think of 'how many people out of 100', or 1,000, or 10,000 – can make a world of difference.

Some great questions you can ask your doctor are:

- Out of 1000 people with this condition, how many will the test detect?
- Of 1000 healthy people who test, how many will be wrongly diagnosed as ill (false positive)?
- Of 1000 sick people who test, how many are wrongly told they are well (false negative)?

If you are basing your medical course of action on the way you understand your probabilities, let's make sure you really understand them. Or at least that you are asking the right questions.

EXERCISE

Has your doc thrown any probabilities, percentages, or stats your way? Write the number you were told (e.g. 3%) at the top of a page in your journal.

Next, **convert it to the frequentist format** (e.g. 3 in 100).

If you can do that, you're all set! But if you find you're still scratching your head, **list a few specific questions** to ask your doctor at your next visit to help you clear things up in your treatment plan (e.g. 'For how many patients out of 1000 will this medication be effective?').

TIPS

Tip 1: Studies show that people do not always base their decisions on medical information and probabilities. You can choose to operate like this, but why not first understand what your chances and risks are, and then you can decide to ignore the stats if you like.

Tip 2: Remember to bring your questions to your next appointment.

Tip 3: Don't be afraid that your doctor will view this as evidence of either mistrust or stupidity. It is neither.

DRIVING HOME THE MESSAGE

Before we delve into this session's topic on interpreting data related to our health, let's have some fun with Art Benjamin, a self-proclaimed "mathemagician." Benjamin is an out-of-the-box college math professor who makes numbers and calculations come alive.

Since understanding statistics can be a crucial aspect of managing your medical condition, let's take some time to take the fear out of numbers and get inspired about their power. So, sit back and enjoy the talk!

Watch 'Faster Than a Calculator' presented by Arthur Benjamin at TEDxOxford on YouTube.

Are stats more important for my health than faith?

Doctors talk in numbers and facts. But how helpful is that from a patient's perspective? Isn't it better to rely on faith, which never lies?

For:

1. By definition, faith is built on that which is unknowable. Numbers are based on fact.
2. No matter how strong your faith is, you have to gather information in order to make sound decisions. You can't just close your eyes and "believe" yourself healthy.
3. Numbers are concrete and can offer you a sense of control.

Add your own argument:

4. _____

Against:

1. There's a certain safety in believing that no matter how things turn out, it was meant to be.
2. Numbers are unreliable. They change the moment new research comes out. My faith is always mine and will remain unchanged no matter who comes out with what shocking new study.
3. Why limit myself to mere statistics? Faith can override any number.

Add your own argument:

4. _____

What's holding you back from understanding your medical condition?

If you don't understand your condition, you won't be able to properly manage it! And yet, there are so many of us who just don't want to understand what's going on… What's holding you back from jumping in?

1. Denial. I'm not really *that* sick, what's there to understand?
2. Inadequacy. I'm just not smart enough to get all this medical mumbo-jumbo.
3. Passivity. I don't need or want to understand. That's what doctors are for.
4. Other commitments. I'm too busy for this!!
5. Contentment. It is what it is. I understand all I need to.
6. Fear. If I realize how sick I am I'll feel much worse.

Add your own:

7. _____

8. _____

9. _____

Take some time brainstorming in your journal about your experience with your medical condition, and then share your story with the Buddy and Soul community! Tag us on Instagram and Twitter @Buddy_N_Soul, using the **#BuddynSoulMedSupport**. By sharing with us on social media, not only can you help others with their personal journeys, you can read about those facing similar challenges.

Getting my medical numbers straight made a huge difference

It's sometimes mind-blowing how understanding something can impact how you relate to it. While getting a grip on the numbers my doctor threw at me didn't *change* my medical condition, it did have a huge impact on how I related to it. Here's how.

What inspires you to understand your medical numbers?

Rethinking how we engage with data is a tall order, but it can be done. If a system doesn't work for you or is confusing, sometimes it just needs to be broken down into numbers. What motivates you to better understand your medical data?

1. Knowledge = power. And a lot of valuable knowledge is to be found in the guise of data and statistics.
2. Overcoming my "statistics allergy" will give me a sense of empowerment and personal growth.
3. Math can be fun, like solving a puzzle. I always love a good challenge.
4. Turning to my number-savvy friends and family gives me an opportunity to get others on board.
5. Numbers can be more telling than abstract concepts. It's worth putting in the effort to understand them properly.

Add your own:

6. _____

7. _____

8. _____

Take some time brainstorming in your journal about your experience with your medical condition, and then share your story with the Buddy and Soul community! Tag us on Instagram and Twitter @Buddy_N_Soul, using the **#BuddynSoulMedSupport**. By sharing with us on social media, not only can you help others with their personal journeys, you can read about those facing similar challenges.

Strategy 4: Get real about your condition

We all like to be perfect. Or, if not perfect, at least we like to ignore our imperfections. A medical condition can be viewed as an imperfection – your body is turning against you, restricting you, and changing your life in ways you do not like and would have wished to avoid. Now what? Some of us choose to soldier on and proceed with denial.

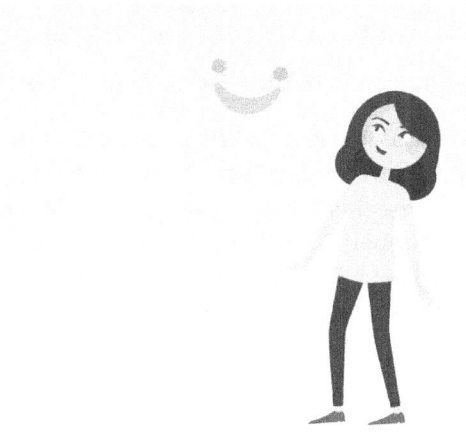

Sometimes our best efforts to protect ourselves and those nearest and dearest to us lead instead to a sense of isolation and our hurting those we love. So who wins?

A Crohn's disease patient, for example, may choose to show up at every family meal not having discussed her dietary needs with her parents, only to be repeatedly disappointed that she's got nothing to eat. A recovering heart patient may show up at a company function only to discover they've planned a competitive team-building activity which would involve far too much exertion for him.

In both cases, proceeding as usual with what others have planned for you would be a mistake. Are you ready to admit, first to yourself, and then to others, that your needs, capabilities, and even priorities, have changed? Doing that takes courage, but can provide relief as well as some very practical help.

Reality might be harsher than you expected. Or brighter. Or just what you suspected. Knowing helps you manage your illness with preparation and astuteness. It also opens up more possibilities for the future.

(Plus: Check out our Defining Your Identity course)

EXERCISE

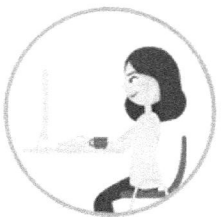

Step 1: **Take the following questionnaire to help determine if you are in medical denial.**

Use your journal to mark each of these statements True or False:

1. Ignorance is bliss. The less I know about my condition, the happier I'll be.
2. I don't want to burden others with my problems, so I under-share.
3. I have a hard time dealing with uncomfortable feelings at the best of times.
4. I'm scared to know the full extent of my 'reality.'
5. I withhold medical information from people I love in order to protect them.
6. Doctors aren't God. What does it matter what they say about my condition?
7. I'm afraid to ask too many questions about my medical condition.

Step 2: **The more Trues you had, the more likely of a candidate you are for medical denial.** You'll want to do some deep introspection and speak to friends and family to ensure you're processing your medical reality in a way that is accurate.

If you had very few Trues, chances are you're on the right track and are able to acknowledge the challenges you're facing. Still, keep an eye out to make sure you continue in this way.

The closer your score was to zero, the more likely it is that you're on the right track and are able to acknowledge the challenges you're facing. Still, keep an eye out to make sure you continue in this way.

TIPS

Tip 1: Knowing doesn't mean succumbing. Get your info right, and then decide what to do about it.

Tip 2: For more on denial and illness check out Emotionally Manage Your Illness.

Tip 3: It is, of course, up to you, to decide to what degree you want to be informed. It's your medical condition.

DRIVING THE MESSAGE HOME

Hey again. Glad you're joining us for our next session.

Today's topic is getting real about your condition. Or in other words, staying positive about your medical condition without denying the realities it entails.

The talk we're about to watch will hopefully serve as a good warm-up for that.

After Janine Shepherd, cross-country skier training for the Olympics, was hit by a truck during a training bike ride and almost died, she describes having an almost surreal out-of-body experience. There she was hovering over her body and debating whether or not it was worth returning to such a body. She describes the crossroads and the choice she made to return to what she viewed as a broken body.

This is a decision many of us battling medical conditions face. How much should we fight for a body that to us seems broken? Do we accept ourselves as we are, limitations and all, or do we choose denial? Shepherd chose to accept herself and her body as it was. Here she tells the tale about the power of the human potential for recovery. Her powerful message: "You are not your body, and giving up old dreams can allow new ones to soar."

Watch 'A Broken Body Isn't a Broken Person' presented by Janine Shepherd at TEDxKC on YouTube.

Does denial serve any good purpose when you're sick?

There are advantages and disadvantages to everything, including denying your medical condition. It's hard to "deny" that when you're sick, denial might actually have some appeal. But is it wise?

For:

1. I'd rather be blissfully asleep than painfully awake, as they say. If denial makes me happy, and living with the reality makes me miserable, what am I gaining?
2. Only in my state of denial can I feel free enough to enjoy the present and to anticipate the future. Otherwise, I'm all doom and foreboding.
3. What denial? I don't have a medical condition.

Add your own argument:

4. _____

Against:

1. Living in a painful reality is infinitely more meaningful than living in an imagined state of bliss.
2. Denial hinders my health. It means I don't take active steps towards managing and improving my condition. I don't want to miss the boat and wake up when it's too late!
3. Though seemingly contradictory, acceptance is a crucial part of my wellbeing. The more I accept, the healthier my mind and body. The more I deny, the more disease festers and proliferates.

Add your own argument:

4. _____

9 Ways denial stops you from managing your condition

There are many obstacles that can prevent you from properly managing your medical condition. Denial is one of the more dangerous ones. Read on and see how denial may be stopping you from successfully managing your condition.
(Plus: Check out our Emotionally Manage Your Illness course)

1. "I'm not really sick." And therefore don't need to go to the doctor.
2. "My meds aren't really helping me." And therefore I don't need to take them.
3. "I know better than my doctor." And therefore don't need to listen to my doctor.
4. "I know smoking/drinking/drug-taking/fill in detrimental behavior here is bad for others. It's not bad for me though." And therefore I can keep up with my bad habit.
5. "I don't eat that much junk food." (Said with a mouth full of chocolate.)
6. "God will take me whenever I'm supposed to go, regardless of what I do now." And therefore I don't need to worry at all about what I do.

Add your own:

7. _____

8. _____

9. _____

How denial held me back from managing my illness

No one wants to believe that their illness is real, or here to stay. But denial isn't the same as hope—it holds you back from proactively managing your condition. Read on to see how denial affected members of the community, and how they dealt with it.

Take some time brainstorming in your journal about your experience with your medical condition, and then share your story with the Buddy and Soul community! Tag us on Instagram and Twitter @Buddy_N_Soul, using the **#BuddynSoulMedSupport**. By sharing with us on social media, not only can you help others with their personal journeys, you can read about those facing similar challenges.

8 Fresh perspectives on accepting your medical condition

It almost feels like accepting your illness means you're giving up, but that's not the case at all. In fact, the more deeply you accept your current situation, the more empowered you'll feel to soldier on with your life and with managing your condition. Here are some thoughts that can help you get there.

1. You can't change the past, but the future is filled with infinite potential. Discovering new possibilities on the horizon can be an exciting journey in and of itself.
2. Taking the straightest route through life might be boring. Twists and turns add a level of excitement and intrigue, always keeping things fresh.
3. Think about all of the things you've learned that you didn't know before. You might even become the go-to expert on your condition, if you haven't already.
4. Your body might have its weaknesses but your spirit is unstoppable.
5. As the famous saying goes, "Whatever doesn't kill you makes you stronger." Find the strength that can be gained from your current circumstances.

Add your own ideas:

6. _____
7. _____
8. _____

Take some time brainstorming in your journal about your experience with your medical condition, and then share your story with the Buddy and Soul community! Tag us on Instagram and Twitter @Buddy_N_Soul, using the **#BuddynSoulMedSupport**. By sharing with us on social media, not only can you help others with their personal journeys, you can read about those facing similar challenges.

Strategy 5: Assume Responsibility

The Internet, and public discourse, are now full of expressions such as patient empowerment, informed patients, e-patients, and what not.

And you?

Are you one of those patients invigorated by the challenge of making a profession out of it, or do you just want to be... plain ol' you?

This is something I've been doing a lot of research on, so buckle up for the ride.
An entire academic movement is dedicated to shared decision making, whereby people are involved in the choices around their care. There is even what we call *The Salzburg Statement on Shared Decision Making*, a declaration born of a convention of all the greatest minds in the field.
Its slogan is "nothing about me without me" ("me" being the patient, of course).
This makes sense and it's even rooted in scientific findings. Because if a patient understands what is being done to her, and even chooses from among various options, she is more likely to adhere to medication, show up to appointments, and feel less conflicted about her care. This has been shown to make a difference in patients who have asthma, cancer, diabetes, hypertension, and patients in end of life situations.

On the other hand, as Harvey Feinberg, head of the Institute of Medicine (IOM) said in response to a paper I wrote (moi! yes!) on shared decision making, it's a patient's right to choose from a menu. And the menu can include shared decision making, informed choice (where the patient makes her own decisions), or good old paternalism, where the doctor makes the decisions for you.

His approach was an interesting wake-up call for me, reminding me not to impose my values and beliefs on other people. He called it patient-centered decision making.

Isn't this what we should strive for in our medical decisions?

EXERCISE

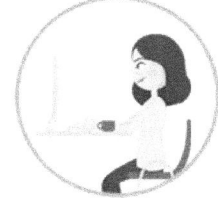

Step 1: **Here are four models of patient care. To what extent do you believe in each?** Write about it in your journal!

- Patient-directed: My physician's role is to rubber-stamp my choices.
- Patient-centered: My physician provides information but I have the final say.
- Shared: I should decide together with my physician.
- Physician-directed: My physician should make all the medical choices.

Step 2: **Does your level of involvement accurately reflect your belief?**

Could it be time to try experimenting with a new model?

Write your thoughts in your journal.

TIPS

Tip 1: There are no rights or wrongs here. The point is that you don't drift into your choices, but rather make them consciously.

DRIVING THE MESSAGE HOME

Tired of waiting at the doctor's office forever? Well, there is hope for change in the future. Watch Eric Topol discuss the latest technological breakthroughs and how, in time, these wireless medical devices will shape the future of medicine for the better.

We no longer need to have a doctor check and monitor us. We can be our own best doctors. As you watch, see how you react to the claim that with the help of technology, we can take responsibility for our health and for the future of our medical conditions.

Watch Eric Topol at TEDMED 2009 on YouTube.

9 Benefits of being an informed patient

As the famous saying goes, "knowledge is power." Here are some great benefits of being more informed when you're managing your medical condition.

1. The more you know, the less surprises you will face along the way.
2. Actually knowing what your doctor is talking about.
3. Feeling more certain. And in this time of uncertainty, this is really calming!
4. Having the ability to preempt issues and plan accordingly
5. Identifying what still remains unknown, and researching those answers.
6. Understanding all treatment options and what comes along with them.

Add your own:

7. _____

8. _____

9. _____

What prevents you from being an informed patient?

Becoming an informed patient is a journey. One that can be smooth or filled with obstacles. What are some of your challenges when trying to become more informed?

1. The medical language is foreign.
2. Time constraints. I'm too busy!
3. Unsupportive family and friends.
4. Unwilling medical staff.
5. Myself.

Add your own:

6. _____

7. _____

8. _____

TAKE A FEW MINUTES AND WRITE IN YOUR COURSE JOURNAL…

I knew I was officially an informed patient when…

It's a wonderful feeling when you sit in front of your doctor and you feel like a peer instead of a lost child. When did you feel informed and in control?

Take some time brainstorming in your journal about your experience with your medical condition, and then share your story with the Buddy and Soul community! Tag us on Instagram and Twitter @Buddy_N_Soul, using the **#BuddynSoulMedSupport**. You can also direct message us YOUR story @Buddy_N_Soul on Instagram and be anonymously featured for a chance to **win a Buddy&Soul three month free membership**. By sharing with us on social media, not only can you help others with their personal journeys, you can read about those facing similar challenges.

Should medicine go wireless?

With technology advancing so rapidly across the board, it won't be long before the entire field of medicine goes completely wireless. But is this a good thing?

For:

1. Imagine the possibilities – remote care, from the comfort of your own home, without the risks of dangerous exposure to other illnesses. Sounds pretty awesome.
2. Wireless systems are not susceptible to human error. A machine will get your dosage right 10 out of 10 times. What a great way to automatically circumvent many of the problems with current healthcare.
3. Wireless technologies placed in the hands of patients is tremendously empowering. We're talking a whole new era of patient-centered care.

Add your own:

4. _____

Against:

1. If there's one field that should never go wireless, it's medicine. We need real-time physicians to be involved in our decisions and care. The risks are just too big.
2. While not susceptible to human error, wireless systems *are* susceptible to hardware and software failures. Who would entrust their health in something so undependable?
3. Patient empowerment is not the bottom line. Better health is. And better health is achieved through joint decision-making with physicians.

Add your own:

4. _____

Strategy 6: Evaluate your choices

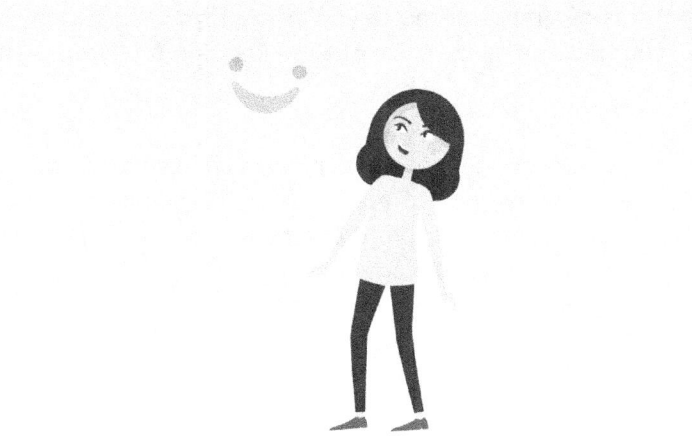

While working on my master's degree in organizational psychology, I ran a project evaluation unit at a large organization. I was amazed to learn how many projects begin and then trail off, or just proceed without anyone determining whether or not they are actually successful.

Once we start doing something, we are likely to continue, for better or for worse. But, are we doing the right thing?

All too often inertia kicks in, as does the fear of finding out we don't like where we're headed and we have toiled in vain. Taking a few more steps in a useless direction is something we've all experienced in the past.

A good way to prevent this from happening is treating each medical course of action as a project: define goals and determine a timetable, budget, milestones, and desired outcomes.

But what about decisions we've made in the past? I can't rewind 10 years and set a retroactive budget and timetable for my meds. So here's another option. Check in with previous medical decisions you've made using these 4 'Re's:

1. **Re-flect**. Reflect on past choices you've made and how they've played out. (E.g. *I chose my current neurologist because she was professional and highly recommended, but I think she might not be the best choice for me after all.*)
2. **Re-evaluate**. Determine what is still working for you and what is not. (E.g. *She and I really don't see eye-to-eye on my treatment plan. I'd like to try switching to someone more open to hearing my concerns.*)
3. **Re-vamp**. Explore alternatives for the choices that you want to redirect. (E.g. *Ask around for new recommendations for a more like-minded neurologist.*)
4. **Re-play**. Implement a change. (E.g. *Make an appointment with a new neurologist.*)

These 4 'Re's are not meant to be a delete button for what you've done previously, but rather, it's a pause button, and then a replay button. It's a way for you to **reflect** back on what was, **reevaluate** if those decisions are still right for you, **revamp** those old decisions to fit with where you are now, and then to **replay** the scenario.

(Plus: Check out our Achieve Your Goals course)

EXERCISE

Think of a medical choice you've made in the past which still has ramifications for your present care. **Write out the decision and your own 4 'Re's below.**

Remember, they are:

1. **Re-flect.** Reflect on the past choice you made and how it has played out.
2. **Re-evaluate**. Determine what is still working for you and what is not.
3. **Re-vamp**. Explore alternatives for redirecting the choice.
4. **Re-play**. Implement a change.

TIPS

Tip 1: You may not be able to replay right away. That's okay. Just knowing that you plan on doing something different in the future helps.

Tip 2: For more on making changes, check out the Tackling Change course.

Tip 3: You may notice, 'regret' is not listed above. And this is for a reason. Don't bash yourself over past mistakes. Just move forward.

DRIVING THE MESSAGE HOME

Great to have you back with us. Now, I'd like to throw a question your way: What's the marker of a well-made medical decision? In today's session, we'll be suggesting that part one of good medical decision-making is making an informed choice – part two is checking in every so often to make sure that the choices you've made in the past are still good for you now.

In the TED Talk we're about to see, Anne Milgram, attorney general of New Jersey, discovered that the criminal justice system was not functioning well; not only did her team not really know who they were putting in jail, but they had no way of understanding if their decisions were actually making the public safer.

Watch her talk and be inspired to make changes when changes are needed! Just because you chose something once, or there's a certain system in place, doesn't mean you're married to it forever.

(Plus: Check out our Tackling Change course)

Watch 'Why Smart Statistics Are the Key to Fighting Crime' presented by Anne Milgram on YouTube.

Is inertia a good guiding principle for managing my condition?

Inertia's basically a fancy way of coasting. Chilling. Letting the tides roll by you. If you ask me, that doesn't sound like an entirely terrible way to manage a medical condition. At least not at first glance…

For:

1. Stress is bad for my medical condition. If more coasting = less stress, count me in.
   (Plus: Check out our Stress Management course)
2. Once I've made a decision, why bother questioning or revisiting it? There are no guarantees that my next decision will lead to better health outcomes.
3. Some call it inertia. Others call it investing in your sanity.

Add your own:

4. _____

Against:

1. I'm changing. Research is changing. My medical condition is changing. My decisions also need to be changing. There is just no room for coasting.
2. The thought of never being able to second guess my initial decision is terrifying. I don't want to be bound by the decisions of my 10-years-younger self.
3. Knowing I always have the right to change my mind takes the pressure and finality off my current decision making.

Add your own:

4. _____

7 Signs you're over-managing your medical condition

Managing your medical condition is crucial. But you know you've taken it too far when…

1. You eat, breathe, and sleep just thinking about your medical condition.
2. Your bathroom reading is medical pamphlets.
3. You have your doctors' numbers on speed dial.
4. You've quit your job in order to find the cure for your medical condition.
5. Your best friends are anonymous people on your medical condition chat line. I mean why bother with old friends? They don't get it anyway.
6. You've asked people to call you by the name of your medical condition. I mean you and it are one, right?
7. You have rated activities according to how good they are for your medical condition. Anything under an eight out of ten you don't bother doing.

Why I decided to switch my course of treatment

Changing a course of treatment is a big deal, and it's not a decision easily made. Share with the community why and how you decided to change your course of treatment, and maybe help others who are coping with similar challenges.

Direct message us YOUR story @Buddy_N_Soul on Instagram and be anonymously featured for a chance to **win a Buddy&Soul three month free membership**. By sharing with us on social media, not only can you help others with their personal journeys, you can read about those facing similar challenges.

12 Reasons to re-evaluate your medical choices

In a fascinating TED Talk, Anne Milgram speaks about the steps she took to make the streets of America a safer place. And guess what. The same steps can be taken towards improving your medical condition. In her opinion, it all boils down to data, research, analytics, and statistics. So, how well-versed were you in the data when you made your latest medical decisions? Here are a few reasons it's worthwhile to revisit past decisions if they were not as informed as they could have been.

1. New research, studies, and data are coming out all the time. You are entitled to change your mind as new information comes to light.
2. Think of yourself as a newbie, no matter how long you've been dealing with anything. Going into something with fresh eyes might give you a different perspective.
3. Even physicians who are top in their field need to go back to basics from time to time. They also need to stay current and up-to-date with the medical advances in their field.
4. Always keep your finger on the pulse of your medical condition. Things change over time and need to be monitored carefully. What worked last year might not be best for you today.
5. Pay as much attention to the information that *isn't* there as to the information that's right in front of you. You might find that you're missing a key piece of the puzzle.
6. View yourself as an outsider looking in. How would you view the options if you were observing someone else being treated for the same thing as you?
7. Don't ignore data and statistics. They can be your window into a world of better health.
8. Employ a broad perspective. Consider the interconnectivity of the body. A medication used to treat one condition might have adverse effects on another part or system of the body.
9. Data and analytics are almost always more accurate than instinct alone. Data is objective and not biased.

Add your own:

10. _____

11. _____

12. _____

Strategy 7: Get your body on track

Up to this point, we've addressed a lot of necessary components to practically manage your medical condition. Now it's time to let your body catch up.

There are so many illnesses out there. And there are exponentially more treatment plans.

However, what most treatment plans seem to have in common is the simultaneous need for generally healthy living.

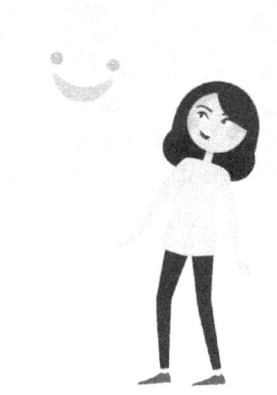

You may not be at a place where you can imagine eating to heal or exercising for fun and yet making proper, balanced lifestyle changes can really contribute to the success of your treatment. **Help your body be the best it can be; you'll only benefit.**

There are studies galore proving the importance of lifestyle in maintaining long-term health. Here are some great examples:

- A team from the University of Toronto's school of medicine researched the amount of time a person sits and exercises every day and the likelihood of developing a chronic disease. Their findings were that there is a direct correlation between daily time spent sitting and risk of heart disease, diabetes, cancer, and death. Among those who exercised in addition, the risk of developing those diseases was lessened.
- A study on mice found that *the offspring* of mice whose mothers exercised regularly during their pregnancy were less likely to develop a neurodegenerative disease than those whose mothers did not.
- In 2009, the American Dietetic Association released a paper stating that well-planned vegetarian diets are not only nutritious for adults, babies and children, but can also help prevent and treat chronic diseases including heart disease, cancer, obesity and diabetes.

So take some time now to help your body to catch up. Creating the right diet and exercise regimens – and sticking with them – makes a big difference in keeping your medical condition stable and in improving your treatment outcome.

EXERCISE

Choose one health-related area (e.g. diet, exercise, sleep, not smoking).

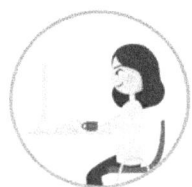

Use your journal to list a few baby steps you could take *this week* that would get you started in the right direction.

To make sure this really happens, also list what will allow you to take each baby step. For example, if you want to get off the subway one stop before your home and walk, you might need to carry comfortable shoes in your bag.

TIPS

Tip 1: Always consult your doctor before beginning an exercise and diet plan!

Tip 2: Commit to a trial period of at least a couple of weeks. Let yourself get used to it and start reaping the benefits. You can always re-evaluate and modify.

Tip 3: Check out our Sleep Well, Spark a Change in Your Eating Habits, and Willpower 101 courses for some more great ideas.

DRIVING THE MESSAGE HOME

Exercise and diet are important factors for managing your medical condition. That's no news. But why is it that for some of us, it's much harder to 'get moving' than for others? According to Emily Balcetis, social psychologist and researcher, the difference is in our minds.

If we think about exercise as difficult, as opposed to easy, it will be much harder for us to start exercising. In fact, according to Balcetis' study, people who are in worse shape see the finish line as further away!

There is a loophole, however. This is only true for people who are not motivated to exercise. Those who have committed to a realistic and manageable goal that they believe they can accomplish regardless of how unfit they were, were much more motivated to exercise and achieve their goal.

This shift in our perspective can be broadened to all things related to our medical condition, and not just exercise. How are you seeing the world through your own mind's eye? Is it positive or negative? Hopeful or bleak?

What changes in your perspective can you make that will increase your motivation to make changes in your life?

Watch 'Why Some People Find Exercise Harder Than Others' presented Emily Balcetis on YouTube.

Isn't my medical treatment infinitely more important than my diet?

Managing my medical condition doesn't leave me with much time or energy for eating wheatgrass and organic kale. Anyway, it's not the main focus here. Is it?

For:

1. I have enough to worry about with my medical condition. I don't need to throw in diet as well.
2. If I give up my comfort foods, what will pick me up when I'm down about my medical condition?
3. People like to point fingers and blame poor health on diet. Well, just because it gives them a focal point and makes them feel better, doesn't mean it's true.

Add your own argument:

4. _____

Against:

1. Diet is one of those magic pills. I know if I improve how I eat, everything else will feel better.
2. Taking care of my lifestyle, including diet and exercise, is a bona fide part of my medical treatment.
3. Ignoring diet as a factor in your health and healing is like brushing your teeth while eating Oreos. Your teeth just won't get clean!
   (Plus: Check out our Spark a Change in Your Eating Habits course)

Add your own argument:

4. _____

How can you take better care of your body?

Having a medical condition can really take a toll on your body. Not to mention, of course, that treatment results are far better when your body is generally healthy and well-maintained. What sort of improvement is your body currently in need of?
(Plus: Check out our Sleep Well and Spark a Change in Your Eating Habits courses)

1. Sleep more
2. Eat better
3. Exercise
4. Get a massage
5. Breathe properly

Add your own:

6. _____

7. _____

8. _____

Take some time brainstorming in your journal about your experience with your medical condition, and then share your story with the Buddy and Soul community! Tag us on Instagram and Twitter @Buddy_N_Soul, using the **#BuddynSoulMedSupport**. By sharing with us on social media, not only can you help others with their personal journeys, you can read about those facing similar challenges.

TAKE A FEW MINUTES AND WRITE IN YOUR COURSE JOURNAL…

What investing in my body did for my condition

Investing in your own body may sound like a scheme, but it does pay off in the end. Read below to see how this investment paid off for others in the community, and add your own story to help inspire others!

Will staying positive impact my health?

In her TED Talk *Why Some People Find Exercise Harder than Others*, social psychologist Emily Balcetis describes the power the mind holds in shaping how we experience the world. Perhaps you're not optimistic about your health because you think it's a lost cause. Will changing your mindset really do anything to improve your health?

(Plus: Check out our Declutter Your Mind course)

For:

1. I don't know if it will or won't heal me, but a positive mindset certainly won't have a *negative* impact on my health. And I think that makes it worth a shot.
2. Actually, many say that a positive attitude *can* improve my health. That's why medical clowns are a growing force to be reckoned with even in the scientific world.
3. There's more to my health than what medications I take. What's going on in my mind impacts the overall picture of my health, including my physical health.

   Add your own argument:

4. _____

Against:

1. It doesn't sound like it will be more successful than all of the other tricks that I've tried.
2. Been there, done that. Didn't work. Moved onto empirically-sound techniques instead.
3. Of course it will take me longer to finish a race than someone who's more toned and in better shape. There's a science to it, just like there's a science to my health.

   Add your own argument:

4. _____

Strategy 8: Forget your condition for a change

When you're managing an illness or a medical condition, it's easy to go overboard.

Rather than creating an isolated "my medical condition" folder in our mental filing cabinet – alongside other folders like "my important relationships," "my life goals," and "what I do for fun" – we often allow all other parts of our life to get pushed aside in favor of our medical concerns.

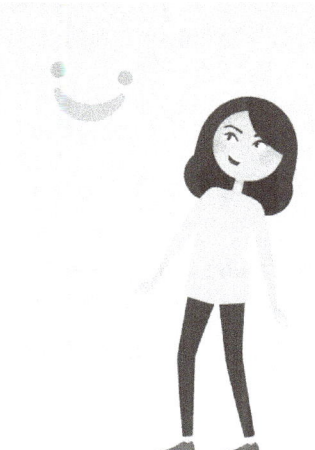

As times goes on, we tend to become more and more entrenched in our anxieties, not less.
In *You Are Not Your Pain* (2015), Burch and Penman explain, "It can seem as if you've always been ill…that you've never found a solution and that you never will. So you can end up being consumed by anxieties, stresses, and worries about the future as well as physical pain" (p. 6).

These anxieties trap us in a vicious downward spiral. They amplify our illness and impair our healing, which in turn leads us to further stress and anxiety (p. 6).

When things go wrong with our life, it is not always because of our illness. And when things go *right*, they shouldn't just be ignored because we are too busy being medical patients.

Whatever we wish to accomplish doesn't dissipate just because we're sick, nor do our past accomplishments.

So let's take some time to draw the illness/non-illness line. Learn to close your medical condition folder every so often and engage other parts of yourself: your career, your hobbies, your ambitions, your relationships…you name it.

Catch a movie, have lunch with a friend, go on a date (or if you're feeling epically brave, a *blind* date), organize your closet, sign up for a parenting course – anything that breaks the cycle and reminds you there's more to you than treatment plans.

Because there's no patient who doesn't deserve at least a *little* time off!
(Plus: Check out our Priorities Reboot course 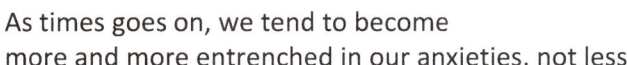)

EXERCISE

Brainstorm as many ideas as you can for ways you could invest in your non-patient self. List them in your journal and then commit to knocking each item off your list – one at a time.

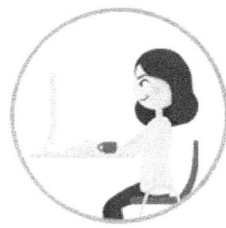

TIPS

Tip 1: If you feel bad taking time and energy away from your medical care – don't! Continuing to live your life will contribute to your sanity and wellbeing – a more-than-worthwhile investment.

Tip 2: You can do a quick online search for ideas and upload a pic here of an activity you plan to pursue.

DRIVING THE MESSAGE HOME

We're about to watch a talk by the talented Patti Dobrowolski – an illustrator who uses art to make change happen. Watch as she demonstrates the power of visuals, and how with one drawing we can transform our lives.

As you watch, think about what you would put in *your* illustration. What would your current state look like, and what would your desired new reality be?

Even if you're working around the clock to manage your medical condition, there's more to you than this illness! Let Dobrowolski's talk inspire you to take three bold steps towards your new, desired reality.

Watch 'Draw Your Future - Take Control of Your Life' presented by Patti Dobrowolski on YouTube.

Can you really 'live your life' when you have a medical condition?

A medical condition is a full-time job...and then some. Who has time to live life after that?

For:

1. Talk about pressure. I'm busy enough as it is!
2. Of course I'll do things I love...after I've kicked this medical condition.
3. If this medical condition has taught me anything, it's to drop all those unnecessary expectations.

Add your own argument:

4. _____

Against:

1. I am not my medical condition. I need to remember that by continuing with my normal, non-illness-related life as much as possible.
2. If I don't live my life, I'll lose my sense of purpose. What am I fighting for, anyway?
3. Effectively managing my medical condition actually gives me more time and energy to live my life.

Add your own argument:

4. _____

11 Out-of-the-box ways to forget illness and live your life

There are some things that might feel a little silly to you. That doesn't matter, as long as it takes your mind off your illness! Tapping into things you haven't done in ages might give you a great feeling of nostalgia. And it's never too late to do something that you've always wanted to do but never found the time for.

1. Learn how to cook a token dish for the next holiday. (Example: Learn how to bake a cake in the shape of a brain for Halloween.)
2. Try an adult coloring book.
3. Find some childhood toys and play with them the way that you used to. If you have kids, bring them on board.
4. It's time to put together that 3000-piece puzzle that you never took out of the box.
5. Go see whatever movie is #1 at the box office. Be generous with yourself at the concession stand.
6. Go on a fun ride. Doesn't matter if it's at an amusement park, or one of those coin operated cars at malls and supermarkets. Make sure to take a picture of yourself doing this.
7. Binge watch an entire TV show season that someone who knows you recommended.
8. Learn a new creative skill like painting or pottery.

Add your own:

9. _____
10. _____
11. _____

Take some time brainstorming in your journal about your experience with your medical condition, and then share your story with the Buddy and Soul community! Tag us on Instagram and Twitter @Buddy_N_Soul, using the **#BuddynSoulMedSupport**. By sharing with us on social media, not only can you help others with their personal journeys, you can read about those facing similar challenges.

TAKE A FEW MINUTES AND WRITE IN YOUR COURSE JOURNAL...

What I focus on to forget my condition

For some, having something to focus on other than their medical condition can be a lifesaver in what is otherwise a stormy sea. Check out what others choose to focus on, and share your own methods of forgetting your condition, if just for a little while.

Take some time brainstorming in your journal about your experience with your medical condition, and then share your story with the Buddy and Soul community! Tag us on Instagram and Twitter @Buddy_N_Soul, using the **#BuddynSoulMedSupport**. By sharing with us on social media, not only can you help others with their personal journeys, you can read about those facing similar challenges.

How Dobrowolski helped me "draw" myself away from my condition

Even if you never thought you were an artist, drawing can be a powerful refuge from the reality of managing a medical condition. Share with the community how Patti Dobrowolski's talk helped you draw away briefly from the reality of managing a medical condition.

Direct message us YOUR story @Buddy_N_Soul on Instagram and be anonymously featured for a chance to **win a Buddy&Soul three month free membership**.

Strategy 9: Get the help you need

Perhaps it's because I'm writing this while visiting England, but the stereotypical stiff upper lip keeps coming to mind. Facing a challenge? Keep calm and carry on. Grin and bear it. Maintain the Blitz spirit.

The world could be falling in on you, but have a cup of tea and don't let on that anything's amiss.

This, however, does not need to be the model we choose when we're in pain or dealing with illness. Being ill is difficult – emotionally, physically, and often also practically.

All those neighbors who rush over with lasagna, chicken soup, chapatti, or casserole (depending on the neighborhood) know what they're doing.

Even if you are the kind of person who prides yourself on independence, illness is a good time to redefine your terms.

You would be surprised what people are willing to do for you. Being an only child, I helped my mother through several hospitalizations. I once saw her through a urine test when she could not get up. It wasn't pretty. The thought of this would likely have horrified her ahead of time, but it happened, and became just one part of the mosaic of our life together.

You will notice that people care and would like to help, but often don't know how. So everyone will come at once, and then you'll have no visitors for days. Or they will buy you expensive flowers, when what you really wanted was for them to pick up your meds and save you a trip to the pharmacy. Even our best-intending friends and relatives are not mind readers, you see.

Don't wait till you feel too bad to ask for help. Don't wait for people to ask, "Why didn't you tell me you needed help?"

Consider what it is you need, and from whom, and reach out.

EXERCISE

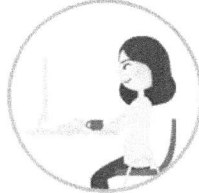

Step 1: **Make a list in your journal of the practical things you cou d really use some help with** – household help, rides, pharmacy runs, etc. Then pair each need with someone you feel could help you.

Step 2: **Do the same with emotional needs.** Whom do you want holding your hand through a frightening procedure, or wiping your tears when you need it, or just being there with you, if you're the strong and silent type?

Finally, don't forget the most important part – reaching out and asking for that help!

TIPS

Tip 1: For more help on the emotional aspect of managing your illness, be sure to check out our course Emotionally Manage Your Illness.

Tip 2: Don't be discouraged if someone says 'no'. It might be that they're busy on a Thursday afternoon, when you need a ride.

Tip 2: Embarrassed to ask for help? Maybe the first bit of help you need is for someone else to be making these calls and inquiries for you.

DRIVING THE MESSAGE HOME

National Geographic writer and explorer Dan Buettner studies the regions of the world with the highest longevity rates, attempting to uncover their secrets for a long, healthy life. One of his projects studies the world's 'Blue Zones,' areas where people live exceptionally long lives. In this TED Talk, he and his team have found secrets that help contribute to a longer life. One, which relates to our session, is social interaction.

With the existence of a positive social peer group, your life expectancy increases by several years. So go out and get the help you need. Share with your loved ones what you are going through with your medical condition, and how they can best support you. Knowing you have somewhere to turn is in itself healing.

Watch 'How to Live to be 100+' presented by Dan Buettner at TEDxTC on www.ted.com.

Can support from others improve my medical condition?

Support from others is great, but it's like icing on the cake. No amount of support can get my medical condition under control. Ultimately, it only comes down to me.

For:

1. It's my family and friends' love and support that helps me through the toughest challenges. And this one is no different.
2. I am definitely not the only one in the world with my particular medical condition. Together, with all of our joint experience, we can bring tremendous comfort, support, and healing to one another.
3. It's my doctors' job to help me with my medical condition. There's no way I can even fathom going it alone.
4. Emotional support is proven to have positive impacts on health and wellbeing! It's far more than just a feel-good bonus.

    Add your own argument:

5. _____

Against:

1. People's support might *feel* good but it won't actually improve my health in any way.
2. I am the one with the medical condition and only I am ultimately responsible for managing it.
3. People can let you down. I can only rely on myself.
4. I hate being a burden on anybody. Even if they *can* help my condition, the price is just too high.

    Add your own argument:

5. _____

What stops you from asking for help when you're sick?

Whether you tend to be more the lone ranger rather or the dedicated group member, the truth is we can all use a little help sometimes. What holds you back from asking for the help you need when you're managing a medical condition?

1. Fear of rejection. What if they say no?
2. Perfectionism. I can do it better myself
3. I really don't need any help
4. I don't want to be a burden
5. Myself

Add your own:

6. _____
7. _____
8. _____

Take some time brainstorming in your journal about your experience with your medical condition, and then share your story with the Buddy and Soul community! Tag us on Instagram and Twitter @Buddy_N_Soul, using the **#BuddynSoulMedSupport**. By sharing with us on social media, not only can you help others with their personal journeys, you can read about those facing similar challenges.

The unlikely place I found help for managing my condition

While having a medical condition is often a lonely journey, it doesn't always have to be. Share with us where you found help, and inspire others to seek help in places they might think unlikely.

Direct message us YOUR story @Buddy_N_Soul on Instagram and be anonymously featured for a chance to **win a Buddy&Soul three month free membership**.

What motivates you to connect with others when you're ill?

In his TED Talk *How to Live to be 100+*, Dan Buettner shows a clear connection between long life and social connections. And yet, for most of us, reaching out is harder than it sounds, especially when we're ill. What motivates you to reach out to others?

1. The research is very compelling and I want to live a long life!
2. I've seen the benefits of social support first-hand.
3. I know that there are greater people than me who have humbled themselves and reached out for support.
4. I know that connection is an irreducible human need. Even if it's awkward, I'll never be satisfied if I am lonely and isolated.
5. Nothing motivates me. I prefer to go it alone.

Add your own:

6. _____

7. _____

8. _____

Strategy 10: Check your checklist

In 2008, the World Health Organization launched an initiative which, though simple and almost childish, they hoped would save thousands of lives around the world every year. And it did.

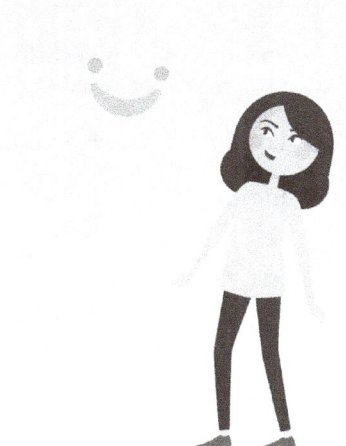

The magic potion? A surgical checklist. The WHO's single-page checklist guides surgical teams through some quick but crucial safety checks before, during, and after performing any operation.

"Whether it's a matter of leaving a sponge inside a patient or failing to ensure sterility, more than 60% of patients worldwide have one of six key safety measures missed during surgery" (WHO, p. 501).

The checklist has significantly decreased human error and improved patient outcomes.

Although they may seem mundane and unnecessary, checklists are empirically-based and have been standardized for use in a number of fields including obstetrics, aviation, marine safety, and even litigation.

So with all this in mind, can you predict how we're about to wrap up our course?

You got it – a checklist.

Your checklist will serve as a summary of everything you've gained from the course from the mission statement in the first session up until this point.

It can be something you check daily, weekly, or monthly – that's up to you. In any case, consider including items that you have difficulty remembering or following through with on your own.

It might end up looking something like this:

- Do I take my meds as required?
- Have I been filling my prescriptions on time?
- Am I spending enough time doing things that bring me joy?
- Is there anything more I can be doing to successfully manage my medical condition?

The idea is to keep it concise so you can run through it quickly and frequently.

You want to make managing your medical condition a habit and way of life.

EXERCISE

Drawing on the goals you've set and the progress you've made throughout the course, it's your turn to **create a checklist.**

What are your criteria for successfully managing *your* medical condition?

Write them out in your journal.

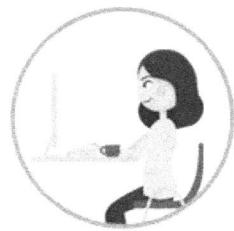

TIPS

Tip 1: Send yourself reminders to check your list regularly!

Tip 2: It's a good idea to check your medical mission statement before you write your checklist.

Tip 3: Your checklist will always be available in your journal for you to review and revise – along with all the other work you've done throughout the course.

DRIVING THE MESSAGE HOME

When you started this course, you created a medical mission statement. To end the course, you're going to be asked to create a checklist you can take with you wherever you go. The purpose of both of these – and everything we've practiced here together – is to help you successfully achieve your goals and effectively manage your medical condition.

To end our course, check out this final TED from Diana Nyad on accomplishing your goals.

Determined to fulfill her lifelong dream of becoming an athlete, she committed herself to an extreme, 100-mile swim from Cuba to Florida. This is the recounting of her journey and how, at age 64, she persevered through a literal sea of obstacles and kept on swimming. Not only is it an incredible story in its own right, it's a constant inspiration for us all to have a dream, no matter how wild it is. To never give up, no matter how challenging it is.

(Plus: Check out our Achieve Your Goals and Priorities Reboot courses)

As you watch, think what you take from her talk and apply to managing your condition, before we wrap up our course.

Watch 'Never Ever Give Up' presented by Diana Nyad at TEDWomen on www.ted.com.

7 Items that don't belong on your medical checklist

A checklist is a great way to help you manage your medical condition, with only one caveat: that what you write on it is relevant. Here are a few ideas of items that do not belong on, or anywhere near, your checklist.

1. *Am I pleasing everyone?* It's *your* health. What other people say, want, or think is *not* your concern. Unless of course they say nice things that make you feel great, in which case, listen to them!
2. *Am I keeping up with my pre-diagnosis standards?* Now that you have a medical condition to manage, it's nearly impossible to maintain the same standards you held before. Loosen your hold in other areas. Your health comes first!
3. *Am I Googling my condition enough?* Don't let the latest and craziest thing you read online mess with your mind and medical management. Is it validated? Credible? Chances are, no. Stick with professional sources.
4. *Am I worrying enough?* You know worrying doesn't help (but if you're worrying, then don't beat yourself up over it).
5. *Am I as informed as a doctor?* Because I could and should be! Well, instead of enrolling in med school, consider building up the connections you already have with your existing medical team. That will greatly improve your chances of effectively managing your condition.
6. *Am I taking every possible precaution?* Take precautions, yes. But no need to go overboard with remote possibilities like the side effect experienced by 1 in a trillion patients that you're sure is coming to get you, even though you have no symptoms of it.
7. *Am I counting my pills every single day?* Now that's just unnecessary. Why you getting all paranoid on us?

Is a medical checklist only for Type A patients?

I'm not a type A person. Why should a method that works for them work for me too? There must be other methods out there that will be a better use of my time and energy. I've got to do what's suited to me and not what works for other people.

For:

1. I say, work with your strengths, not against them. Pushing myself into a poor-fitting box will just make me feel inadequate and on edge.
2. If I'm already going to push myself beyond my comfort zone, there are more important things I'd rather do than create a personal medical checklist.
3. Yes. That's why there are programs and apps for the rest of us.

Add your own argument:

4. _____

Against:

1. If it works for Type A people, then why shouldn't it work for me too?
2. Type A people are really good at getting stuff done. I can learn from them. Who cares whether or not it comes naturally?
3. I'm sure my medical professional would recommend this method. And that's enough motivation for me!

Add your own argument:

4. _____

TAKE A FEW MINUTES AND WRITE IN YOUR COURSE JOURNAL…

How a checklist improved my health

Sometimes big ideas come in somewhat mundane packages. Here's how something as simple as a checklist helped me improve my health, even if it was in a somewhat roundabout way!

TAKE A FEW MINUTES AND WRITE IN YOUR COURSE JOURNAL...

The near-impossible health goal I set, and accomplished!

It may have seemed impossible at first, but you've achieved a goal that seemed totally out of reach! Share with the community what your goal was, and how you reached it despite any difficulties that may have arisen along the way.

Direct message us YOUR story @Buddy_N_Soul on Instagram and be anonymously featured for a chance to **win a Buddy&Soul three month free membership**.

WHERE DO WE GO FROM HERE?

You've finished the Manage Your Medical Condition book, but you haven't finished the journey. It doesn't end, it just gets better. Revisit this book, carry its ideas with you. Check out BuddynSoul.com and the rest of our books for all we have to offer. Spread the word. And change your life for good.

Create a Pleasant Reality

Whether you've found yourself struggling with depression or are just looking to make your day-to-day life more enjoyable, this book is for you. We've created this book as a multimedia tool for you to learn how to create a pleasant reality. You can do it. And we all need it.

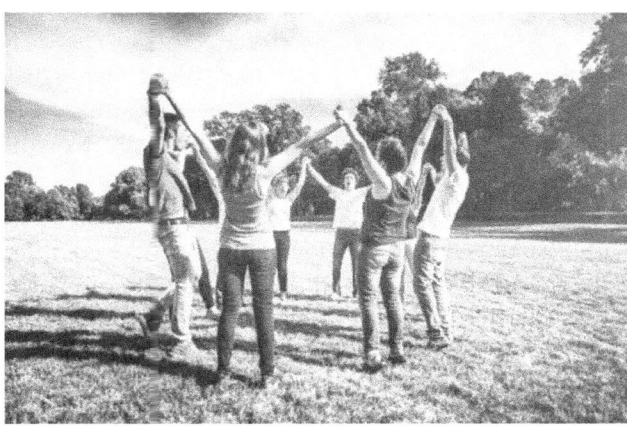

Goals you can achieve by reading 'Create a Pleasant Reality':

1. Understand what holds you back from enjoying life.
2. Learn tools to change the things you can and embrace the things you can't.
3. Tap into the power of ordinary moments to add joy and meaning to your life.

Emotionally Managing your Illness

Being ill is not easy. A lot is going on, and very little of it is fun. Being asked "how are you feeling?" might be nice the first few thousand times, but eventually it seems either redundant (I feel terrible! Still! But thanks for asking…) or like a sham (I'm falling apart at the seams, but I'll beam a smile and say "fine" because I don't have the energy to entertain pity). It may also seem beside the point, because you are ill, physically unwell, so what else is there to know? But, connecting with how you feel is actually one of the most important parts of having and managing a disease.

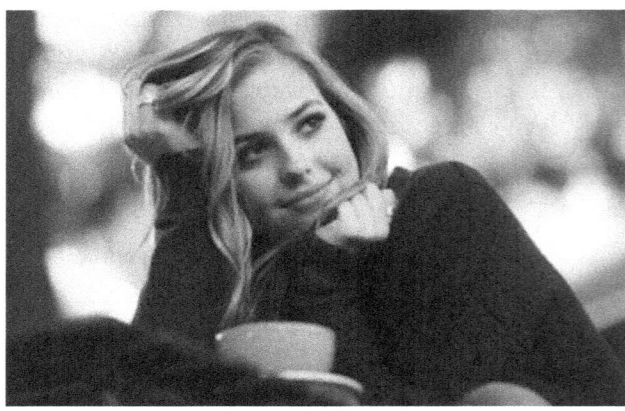

Goals you can achieve from reading 'Emotionally Managing Your Illness':
1. Identify, map out and sort your feelings regarding your illness.
2. Find strength and emotional balance to see you through your medical condition.
3. Take responsibility for your emotional well-being during your illness.

Adhering to Your Medication

Taking your medication is vital, especially when it comes to optimizing your long-term health. And yet, if you're taking this course, you know how hard it is to take your medication in a timely and efficient manner. And to do it all the time! This course offers you a fresh new look into adhering to your medication by exploring the cognitive, emotional, and behavioral elements that may be preventing you from improving your medication adherence, and your health outcomes.

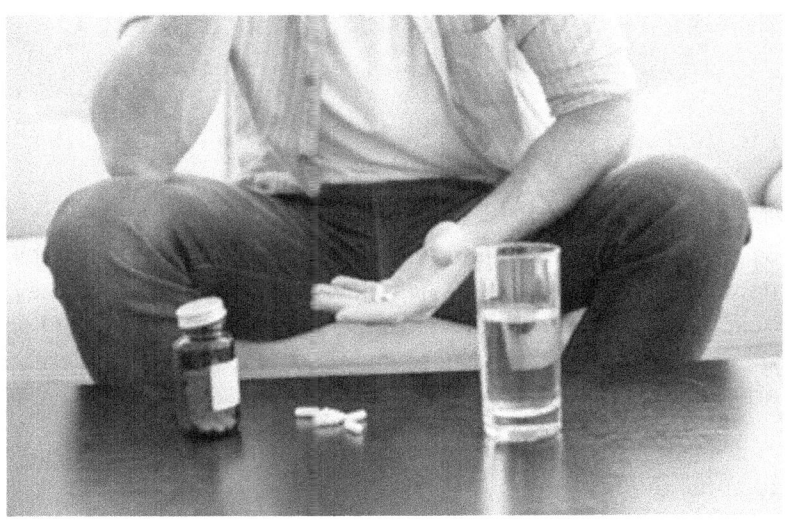

Goals you can achieve from reading 'Adhering to your Medication':

1. Delve a little deeper into what may be holding you back from optimal adherence.
2. Learn practical tools to help ensure you take your meds as needed.
3. Assume responsibility for how you handle adherence to medication.

WANT TO LEARN MORE? CHECK THESE OUT!

MOVIES

Garden State (2004)

Sam (who has epilepsy) and Andrew (who has taken mood stabilizers for many years) meet at a neurologist's office. The movie follows Sam and Andrew as they get to know and trust each other and build a relationship. When Sam shares with Andrew some of her personal life challenges, Andres learns the value of allowing himself to identify and experience his emotional world – even when the emotions are not pleasant.

This movie explores how much you need to *feel* when managing your medical condition, and is it ever too much?

Jack (1996)

Jack Powell has Progeria and Werner Syndrome (an aging disease) – a condition that gives him the appearance of a 40-year old man when he is only 10. His parents, trying to protect him, keep him homeschooled and isolated. Fed up, Jack decides to venture into the real world by going to public school to make friends of his own. Being exposed to real life allows Jack to experience the fullness of his emotional realm as well as the limitations of his illness.

While his disease is rare, anyone managing a medical condition has felt isolated at times. Let this movie remind you that even if you're alone in your disease, you don't have to be lonely.

MORE VIDEOS

Sam Berns, My philosophy for a happy life, TEDxMidAtlantic

Sam Berns was diagnosed with Progeria, a rare, rapid-aging disease, before he was 2 years old. His family started the Progeria Research Foundation in order to increase awareness of the disease, provide support for family members of those suffering from Progeria, and to provide funding for research for a cure. His life story can be watched in the documentary *Life According to Sam*. Watch him share his philosophy for a happy life.

Alison Ledgerwood, Getting stuck in the negatives (and how to get unstuck), TEDxUCDavis

Do you want to work on managing your illness, but keep getting stuck in your own negative thoughts? Watch this great TED Talk by Alison Ledgerwood, professor in the Department of Psychology at UC Davis, discussing research that shows we can get unstuck in our negative thoughts.

BOOKS

Undone: A Story of Making Peace with an Imperfect Life, by Michele Cushatt

Michele Cushatt's memoir faces her cancer diagnosis head on. Suddenly charged with the task of making peace with a very complicated life, she starts weighing her past and future as her need for control takes over.
It's through living in the day-to-day moments that she becomes aware of what life is really all about, despite and *because* of her medical condition.

The Anatomy of Hope – How You Can Find Strength in the Face of Illness, by Jerome E. Groopman

A physician and patient himself, Jerome Groopman discusses the importance of hope in the face of illness.

Regardless of diagnosis and prognosis, it is hope that triumphs time and time again over the emotional and physical aspects of disease.

GADGETS AND PRODUCTS

My Health, A Medical Records Journal - Kraft Hard Cover

This medical journal is a great way to get motivated to write about managing your medical condition. It provides prompts on every page to write about your symptoms, feelings, and doctors' recommendations.

Personal Health Record Keeper and Logbook

This personal record keeper allows you to keep all your important medical information in your bag at all times. It has designated spaces for your personal profile (i.e. blood type, allergies, etc.), insurance and pharmacy information, doctors' and specialists' information, family health history, and much more.

www.ingramcontent.com/pod-product-compliance
Lightning Source LLC
Chambersburg PA
CBHW060434220526
45465CB00008B/3141